THE EMPOWERED SEX GUIDE FOR WOMEN

Unlocking Self-Awareness and Deepening Intimacy

Ethan Wellspring

Contents

Ethan Wellspring

Ethan Wellspring

Introduction

Imagine living in a world where your desires are not just understood, but celebrated. Where your body is not a mystery to solve, but a source of power, pleasure, and confidence. The Empowered Sex Guide for Women: Unlocking Self-Awareness and Deepening Intimacy isn't just another book about sex—it's a key to unlocking a more authentic, empowered version of yourself. It's time to rewrite the narrative of female sexuality, one that embraces self-discovery, deep intimacy, and unapologetic confidence.

For far too long, society has dictated what women should and shouldn't desire. We've been conditioned to silence our needs, to carry shame about our bodies, and to accept a shallow version of intimacy. But now, a new chapter begins—one where you, as a woman, take full control of your sexual identity, breaking free from myths and discovering what truly makes you feel alive.

This guide is different. It's not about learning to please others; it's about you. It's about gaining a deeper understanding of your body, your pleasure, and your

Ethan Wellspring

power. It's about creating intimate, meaningful connections—whether with yourself or a partner—that are rooted in mutual respect, trust, and excitement.

You may have questions about your sexual identity that you've been afraid to ask. You might be yearning for a deeper connection in your relationship but don't know how to get there. Or maybe you simply want to feel more confident in your skin, fully embracing your body's unique desires. Wherever you are on your journey, this book will take you further.

Through practical steps, expert insights, and real-world stories, The Empowered Sex Guide for Women is your blueprint to understanding your body in ways you never thought possible. You'll learn how to connect with your desires without shame, how to confidently communicate with your partner about what truly excites you, and how to create lasting intimacy that fulfills both body and soul.

But this isn't just about sex. It's about empowerment in every sense of the word. When you are fully in tune with your sexual self, that confidence spills over into all areas of life—your career, your relationships, your mental and

Ethan Wellspring

emotional well-being. This is about embracing a holistic sense of wellness that comes from truly knowing yourself, inside and out.

This guide will challenge the status quo. It will ask you to leave behind the limitations society has placed on female sexuality and step into a space where pleasure, self-awareness, and intimate connection are your birthright. Whether you're reclaiming your sexual power or exploring it for the first time, this book will equip you with the tools, knowledge, and confidence to transform your relationship with your body and your partners.

Are you ready to dive deeper? To explore your desires fearlessly, and build a life of intimacy, empowerment, and fulfillment? Welcome to your sexual revolution. Your journey starts here.

Ethan Wellspring

Chapter 1: Understanding Sexual Self-Awareness

What Is Sexual Self-Awareness?

Sexual self-awareness is the foundation of a fulfilling and meaningful sex life. But what does it truly mean? It's the conscious understanding of your own sexual identity—your needs, desires, limits, and boundaries. It involves introspection and reflection on how you feel about sex, how your body responds, and how your emotional and mental states influence your experiences in the bedroom. Sexual self-awareness transcends just knowing what turns you on; it's about being in tune with your emotions, body, and thoughts, and how they all intertwine during intimacy.

For many, this level of self-awareness may seem elusive or unfamiliar due to societal conditioning, cultural taboos, or personal insecurities. We've often been taught to view our sexuality through a limited or distorted lens, but breaking free from these perspectives is the first step toward reclaiming your sexual identity.

Ethan Wellspring

Understanding your own sexual self-awareness empowers you to:

- Clearly articulate what you want in intimate situations.
- Set personal boundaries with confidence and without guilt.
- Develop a deeper connection to your body, fostering greater pleasure and satisfaction.

In the coming pages, we will explore not only how to cultivate this self-awareness but also how to apply it practically in your relationships and solo experiences. By the end of this chapter, you will have the tools to dive deeper into your sexual identity and communicate your desires with clarity and confidence.

Exploring Your Desires and Boundaries

To truly embrace sexual self-awareness, it's vital to reflect on your desires and boundaries. Sexual desires are often

Ethan Wellspring

fluid, evolving over time based on experiences, emotional shifts, and external influences. It's common for people to suppress or ignore their desires due to fear of judgment, guilt, or cultural conditioning. However, fully embracing and understanding what you want is key to achieving sexual satisfaction.

Reflection Exercises to Explore Your Desires:

- **Quiet Reflection:** Take some time to sit quietly with your thoughts. Ask yourself questions like: What kind of touch do I enjoy? What are my fantasies? Are there certain activities that I've always been curious about but never explored? Let your mind wander without judgment.

- **Journaling:** Write down your thoughts on past sexual experiences—both positive and negative. Reflect on what made the good experiences enjoyable and why the bad ones weren't fulfilling. This can help you clarify what works for you and what doesn't.

Ethan Wellspring

- **Visualization:** Picture an ideal sexual encounter. What does it look like? What do you feel emotionally and physically? How does your partner (if any) respond? Visualization can help you tap into desires you may not have previously considered.

Once you've explored your desires, it's just as important to establish and understand your boundaries. Boundaries protect your emotional and physical well-being, allowing you to engage in sexual experiences that feel safe and enjoyable. Boundaries can evolve, but knowing where you stand at any given moment is crucial.

Setting Boundaries:

- **Physical Boundaries**: These define what kinds of touch you are comfortable with. This could involve certain areas of your body that are off-limits or activities that make you uncomfortable.

- **Emotional Boundaries**: Emotional boundaries help you protect your mental and emotional state

Ethan Wellspring

during and after sexual experiences. For example, you may not be comfortable with certain discussions or situations post-intimacy, and that's okay.

- **Communicating Boundaries:** Knowing your boundaries is one thing—communicating them is another. Learning to articulate them in a calm, clear, and honest manner is essential for maintaining a healthy sexual dynamic with your partner.

The Role of Body Positivity in Sexual Confidence

Your relationship with your body plays a significant role in your sexual self-awareness. How you perceive your body can either enhance or diminish your sexual confidence. Society often perpetuates unrealistic beauty standards, leaving many women to feel inadequate or ashamed of their bodies. This shame can manifest in the bedroom, causing discomfort, hesitation, or avoidance of intimacy altogether.

Ethan Wellspring

Body positivity is about embracing your body as it is, appreciating its uniqueness, and celebrating its strength and beauty. When you foster a positive body image, you open yourself up to deeper, more fulfilling sexual experiences. But achieving body positivity doesn't happen overnight. It requires conscious effort, patience, and sometimes a change in perspective.

Steps to Cultivating Body Positivity:

- **Shift Your Perspective**: Instead of focusing on your perceived flaws, start viewing your body as a source of pleasure, strength, and beauty. Celebrate what your body can do—its ability to feel, to give pleasure, and to move in ways that make you feel alive.

- **Affirmations**: Practice positive self-talk. Instead of criticizing your body, speak kindly to yourself. For example, say things like "I love the way my body responds to touch" or "My body is beautiful just

Ethan Wellspring

the way it is." Over time, these affirmations can help rewire your thinking.

- **Surround Yourself with Positivity:** The people and media you expose yourself to play a huge role in shaping your body image. Seek out body-positive communities, follow influencers who celebrate diversity in body types, and avoid media that perpetuates harmful beauty standards.

- **Mindfulness**: Pay attention to how your body feels in the moment. Engage in mindful activities, such as yoga, dance, or even simple stretching exercises, that encourage you to connect with your body without judgment. Mindfulness can help you become more attuned to your body's sensations, increasing sexual confidence.

By learning to love and appreciate your body, you can approach sex with a sense of ease and confidence, enhancing not only your self-awareness but also your sexual satisfaction.

Ethan Wellspring

In this chapter, we've laid the groundwork for sexual self-awareness by defining the concept, encouraging exploration of desires and boundaries, and discussing the pivotal role body positivity plays in sexual confidence. As you move forward, remember that understanding yourself sexually is an ongoing journey. It requires introspection, compassion for yourself, and the willingness to push past societal expectations. By nurturing this awareness, you will not only enhance your sexual experiences but also improve your overall relationship with yourself and others.

Ethan Wellspring

Chapter 2: The Female Body and Sexual Response

Anatomy 101: Knowing Your Body

Understanding the female body is an essential part of sexual self-awareness and satisfaction. Female anatomy is often underexplored or misunderstood, even by women themselves. Yet, learning about your body's structure and its erogenous zones can significantly improve your sexual experiences. By becoming familiar with your body, you not only boost your sexual confidence but also empower yourself to communicate better with your partner.

Let's break down the key components of female anatomy in a straightforward manner:

- **The Vulva**: The vulva includes the external parts of the female genitalia. This includes the labia (both majora and minora), the clitoris, the urethral

Ethan Wellspring

opening, and the vaginal opening. Each part plays a unique role in sexual pleasure and response.

- **Clitoris:** The clitoris is packed with thousands of nerve endings, making it one of the most sensitive areas on a woman's body. It's crucial to understand that the clitoris extends internally as well, meaning stimulation isn't confined just to the external part you see.

- **The Vagina**: The vagina is the muscular canal that connects the external genitals to the cervix and uterus. While many focus solely on penetration, the vagina has many sensory receptors that can be responsive to stimulation, particularly around the vaginal opening.

- **The G-Spot**: Located a few inches inside the vagina on the front wall, the G-spot is another erogenous zone that can bring intense pleasure when stimulated. However, its sensitivity can vary from woman to woman, so exploration is key to discovering your preferences.

Ethan Wellspring

- **The Breasts:** Breasts, and more specifically nipples, are another highly sensitive area. Like the clitoris, the nipples contain a large concentration of nerve endings that can trigger pleasurable sensations when stimulated.

- **Other Erogenous Zones:** Beyond the genitals and breasts, the body has numerous erogenous zones, such as the neck, ears, inner thighs, and even the lower back. Each woman is different, so take time to explore and find out what works best for you.

Familiarity with these parts of your body is not just about anatomy but also about connection. The more you understand how your body works, the more confident you'll feel in seeking and communicating what brings you pleasure.

The Science of Arousal

Arousal is a complex interplay between the brain, emotions, hormones, and physical responses. It's not just about physical stimulation but also about the mental and

Ethan Wellspring

emotional state you're in. The mind is often considered the most powerful sexual organ, as it influences how your body reacts to stimuli.

Let's break down how sexual arousal works:

- **Hormones and Chemistry:** The brain releases various hormones, including dopamine (the "feel-good" hormone) and oxytocin (the "bonding" hormone), which play pivotal roles in the arousal process. These chemicals create feelings of excitement, connection, and pleasure, which can enhance your physical responses.

- **Physical Response:** As the brain sends signals to the body, the physical signs of arousal begin to appear—such as increased heart rate, faster breathing, and genital lubrication. Blood flows to the genitals, causing the clitoris and vulva to become engorged, which makes them more sensitive to touch.

Ethan Wellspring

- **The Role of the Mind:** Mental and emotional factors heavily influence sexual arousal. For many women, the mind must be fully engaged for their bodies to reach full arousal. This is why emotional connection and mental stimulation (fantasy, for example) are often critical components of sexual satisfaction.

- **The Role of Emotions**: Emotional intimacy and comfort also play a large part in arousal. Feeling secure and connected to your partner can lower inhibitions and increase the ease of becoming aroused. In contrast, stress, anxiety, or unresolved emotional issues can inhibit arousal, regardless of physical stimulation.

- **The Plateau of Arousal**: Once aroused, your body may enter a plateau phase, where excitement and sensitivity peak, and you feel close to orgasm. Learning to recognize this phase can help prolong the pleasurable sensations and prepare for orgasm.

By understanding how your mind and body work together to create arousal, you can learn to enhance your experiences, making them more satisfying. This knowledge also equips you to better communicate with your partner, ensuring that your needs are understood and met.

Understanding Your Sexual Response Cycle

The sexual response cycle is a series of stages your body and mind go through during sexual activity. Knowing these stages can help you better understand your body's signals and improve your sexual experiences. The sexual response cycle includes four distinct phases:

- **Excitement**: This phase begins with the initial feelings of sexual arousal. Your heart rate increases, blood flow to the genitals intensifies, and you may begin to feel warm or flushed. For women, the clitoris swells, and lubrication increases in preparation for intercourse.

Ethan Wellspring

- **Plateau:** During this phase, arousal continues to build. Sensitivity to touch is heightened, and muscles throughout your body begin to tense in anticipation of orgasm. Your breathing becomes faster, and your body prepares for the peak of pleasure.

- **Orgasm:** The climax of the sexual response cycle, orgasm is marked by a release of tension built up during the excitement and plateau phases. It involves rhythmic contractions of the pelvic muscles and a surge of pleasurable sensations. The intensity and duration of an orgasm can vary from person to person and from experience to experience.

- **Resolution:** After orgasm, the body begins to relax and return to its normal state. Blood pressure and heart rate drop, and the genitals return to their unaroused state. During this phase, many women feel a deep sense of relaxation or satisfaction.

Understanding these stages helps you recognize where you are during sexual activity and enables you to prolong or

Ethan Wellspring

enhance certain phases for more satisfying experiences. For instance, if you're aware that you're in the plateau stage, you can communicate with your partner to maintain this heightened state longer, intensifying your eventual orgasm.

Knowledge is empowerment. By understanding the complexities of the female body, the science of arousal, and the sexual response cycle, you can unlock new levels of sexual satisfaction and confidence. Remember, every woman's experience is unique, so it's essential to explore your own responses and preferences. As you delve deeper into understanding your body and sexual responses, you'll find that the more connected you are to yourself, the more fulfilling your sexual experiences will be.

Ethan Wellspring

Chapter 3: Overcoming Sexual Shame and Taboos

Breaking Free from Cultural and Social Barriers

Sexual shame is a pervasive issue that many women face, often stemming from cultural and societal expectations. These influences can create feelings of guilt or embarrassment around natural desires and behaviors, significantly impacting sexual confidence and fulfillment.

The Origins of Sexual Shame:

- o Sexual shame can be traced back to various cultural, religious, and familial teachings that promote the idea that female sexuality is something to be suppressed or controlled. These beliefs can create an internalized sense of shame that hinders sexual exploration and enjoyment.
- o Understanding the origins of this shame can be the first step in dismantling it. Many women may

Ethan Wellspring

find comfort in sharing their experiences with others who have faced similar societal pressures.

Challenging Societal Norms:

- o By questioning the societal narratives that dictate how women should view their sexuality, we can begin to reclaim our sexual agency. This involves recognizing that pleasure is not only natural but is also a vital aspect of human experience.
- o Engaging with communities or movements that advocate for sexual liberation can provide support and validation. These groups often work to reshape the conversation around female sexuality, challenging harmful stereotypes and promoting a more inclusive understanding.

Personal Reflection and Growth:

- o Engaging in self-reflection can help identify the specific beliefs that contribute to feelings of shame. Journaling, therapy, or discussions with trusted friends can be valuable tools for exploring these feelings.

Ethan Wellspring

- o Creating a personal narrative that embraces sexuality can empower women to take control of their experiences. This may involve reframing thoughts and beliefs about sexuality as positive, liberating, and worthy of exploration.

Addressing Common Sexual Myths

Many misconceptions about female sexuality perpetuate shame and hinder confidence. Debunking these myths is essential to promoting a healthier understanding of sexual experiences.

> **Myth #1: Women Shouldn't Enjoy Sex as Much as Men:**

This myth has historical roots in patriarchal societies that have often portrayed female pleasure as secondary to male desire. In reality, women are equally capable of enjoying sex, and acknowledging this can be empowering.

> **Myth #2: Orgasm Is the Ultimate Goal of Sex:**

While orgasm can be a pleasurable aspect of sexual experiences, it is not the only measure of success. Many women find intimacy, connection, and exploration to be equally satisfying.

Understanding that sexual experiences can be fulfilling without the pressure to achieve orgasm can lead to more relaxed and enjoyable encounters.

Myth #3: It's Normal for Women to Have Low Libido:

The idea that women naturally have a lower sex drive than men is not universally true. Libido is influenced by numerous factors, including physical health, emotional state, and relationship dynamics.

Encouraging open dialogue about desires and needs can help dispel this myth and foster a more accurate understanding of individual sexual appetites.

Reclaiming Your Sexual Narrative

Empowerment comes from taking ownership of your sexual story. Reclaiming your narrative involves

Ethan Wellspring

understanding your desires and making choices that reflect your values and needs.

Writing Your Own Story:

- Begin by articulating what sexuality means to you. What are your desires, boundaries, and preferences? Journaling can be an effective way to explore these thoughts and gain clarity on your sexual identity.
- Share your narrative with others who support and uplift you. This can foster a sense of community and validation as you navigate your sexual journey.

Redefining Sexuality:

- Understand that your sexual identity is uniquely yours. There is no one-size-fits-all approach to sexuality, and embracing your individuality can liberate you from societal expectations.
- Celebrate your journey of self-discovery. Each experience, whether positive or negative, contributes to your understanding of yourself and your sexuality.

Ethan Wellspring

Setting Boundaries:

- Establishing and communicating personal boundaries is crucial for sexual health and satisfaction. Know what you are comfortable with and assert these boundaries in your relationships.
- Empowering yourself to say "no" when necessary is a vital part of reclaiming your sexual narrative. This not only protects your well-being but also reinforces your right to determine your own sexual experiences.

Overcoming sexual shame and taboos requires courage and commitment. By breaking free from cultural barriers, debunking harmful myths, and reclaiming your sexual narrative, you can foster a more fulfilling and confident sexual identity. Remember, you are not alone in this journey. Engaging with supportive communities and advocating for your needs can lead to profound personal growth and empowerment.

Ethan Wellspring

Ready to continue this transformative journey? Let's move on to Chapter 4: Communication and Intimacy in Relationships.

Ethan Wellspring

Ethan Wellspring

Chapter 4: Communication and Intimacy in Relationships

The Art of Open and Honest Sexual Communication

Effective communication is the cornerstone of any healthy relationship, especially when it comes to sexual intimacy. Open dialogue about desires, boundaries, and preferences can foster a deeper connection between partners.

Creating a Safe Space for Dialogue:

- Establish an environment where both partners feel comfortable discussing their sexual needs without fear of judgment. This may involve setting aside dedicated time for these conversations, free from distractions.
- Use "I" statements to express feelings and desires. For example, saying "I feel more connected when we explore new things

Ethan Wellspring

together" is more constructive than "You never want to try anything new."

Being Vulnerable:

- Sharing personal desires and fears can deepen emotional intimacy. Vulnerability encourages partners to engage with each other on a more profound level, enhancing both sexual and emotional connections.
- Acknowledge that it's okay to feel nervous or uncertain when discussing sensitive topics. Approach these conversations with compassion and patience, both for yourself and your partner.

Regular Check-ins:

- Sexual preferences can evolve over time, making it essential to have ongoing conversations about intimacy. Regularly check in with your partner about what feels good and what may need to change.
- Encourage feedback and be open to discussing what each partner enjoys or finds challenging. This ongoing dialogue can help prevent misunderstandings and keep the relationship dynamic.

Ethan Wellspring

Creating Emotional and Sexual Intimacy

Emotional intimacy lays the groundwork for a fulfilling sexual relationship. When partners feel emotionally connected, they are often more comfortable exploring physical intimacy.

Building Emotional Connection:

- Spend quality time together, engaging in activities that foster connection, whether through deep conversations, shared hobbies, or simply enjoying each other's company.
- Practice empathy and understanding. Make an effort to listen actively to your partner's thoughts and feelings, validating their experiences and emotions.

Physical Affection Beyond Sex:

- Engage in non-sexual physical touch, such as cuddling, holding hands, or gentle massages. These forms of affection can strengthen your

Ethan Wellspring

bond and create a safe atmosphere for sexual exploration.

- Understand that intimacy doesn't always have to lead to sex. Cultivating a close relationship outside of sexual encounters can enhance sexual experiences when they do occur.

Exploring Intimacy Through Shared Experiences:

- Engage in new experiences together, whether trying a new activity, taking a class, or exploring a new place. Shared experiences can create lasting memories and strengthen emotional intimacy.
- Consider taking a relationship or intimacy workshop together. These experiences can provide tools and insights that enhance both emotional and sexual intimacy.

Navigating Differences in Libido and Desires

It's common for partners to experience mismatched libidos or differing sexual desires. Navigating these differences

Ethan Wellspring

requires understanding, patience, and effective communication.

Recognizing Normal Variability:

- Understand that sexual desire fluctuates for everyone due to various factors, including stress, hormonal changes, and life circumstances. Recognizing that fluctuations are normal can ease tension around the subject.
- Avoid making assumptions about your partner's desires or motivations. Openly discussing feelings can help clarify any misconceptions.

Finding Compromise:

- Approach discussions about libido differences with a mindset of collaboration. Work together to find solutions that honor both partners' needs and desires.
- Explore options such as scheduling intimate time together or engaging in other forms of intimacy when one partner may not feel up to sexual activity.

Ethan Wellspring

Seeking Professional Help:

- If differences in libido become a source of conflict, consider seeking guidance from a sex therapist or relationship counselor. These professionals can provide strategies for navigating mismatches in desire while promoting understanding and intimacy.
- Workshops or counseling can also offer practical tools to help partners communicate effectively and find common ground.

The foundation of a fulfilling sexual relationship lies in open and honest communication, emotional connection, and a willingness to navigate differences together. By fostering a safe environment for dialogue and embracing vulnerability, partners can deepen their intimacy and create a more satisfying sexual relationship.

With this understanding, let's move on to Chapter 5: Empowering Solo Exploration.

Ethan Wellspring

Chapter 5: Empowering Solo Exploration

In the journey of understanding and embracing one's sexuality, solo exploration stands as a powerful and essential practice. It serves not only as a source of pleasure but also as a means of self-discovery, empowerment, and intimacy with oneself. By nurturing this connection with our bodies, we pave the way for a more fulfilling sexual experience both solo and with partners.

The Importance of Self-Exploration

Self-exploration is a fundamental aspect of sexual self-awareness. It allows individuals to cultivate a deeper understanding of their bodies and desires. Masturbation and solo play, often stigmatized, are natural and healthy practices that can significantly enhance sexual well-being.

The act of exploring one's body can yield profound benefits. Physically, it helps individuals learn about what

Ethan Wellspring

feels pleasurable, paving the way for better sexual experiences. Psychologically, it contributes to increased body confidence and a positive self-image. Moreover, by engaging in self-exploration, individuals can reduce anxiety related to sexual performance and open the door to a more liberated expression of their sexuality.

Despite the cultural taboos surrounding solo exploration, it is essential to approach it with an open mind. Embracing the practice can lead to greater self-acceptance and the realization that pleasure is a personal journey, unique to each individual.

Tools and Techniques for Solo Pleasure

Equipped with an understanding of its importance, we can now explore various tools and techniques that can enhance solo sexual experiences.

First and foremost, sex toys have revolutionized the way individuals engage in self-exploration. From vibrators to dildos, there is an array of options designed specifically for female pleasure. The key is to find the right tools that

Ethan Wellspring

resonate with personal preferences. Trying different types of toys can be a fun and liberating experience, allowing for the exploration of various sensations and techniques.

For those who prefer a more hands-on approach, learning specific techniques can elevate the experience. Techniques may include experimenting with different types of touch, such as varying pressure, speed, and rhythm. Guided fantasies, whether through erotic literature, podcasts, or films, can help set the mood and ignite the imagination, leading to a more fulfilling experience.

Creating the right environment is equally crucial. Setting the mood can greatly enhance the overall experience. Consider dimming the lights, playing soft music, or using aromatherapy to create a sensual atmosphere. Allowing oneself to be fully present during the experience without distractions is vital to embracing the moment.

Ethan Wellspring

Building a Healthy Relationship with Your Sexual Self

The journey of self-exploration is also about nurturing a positive relationship with one's body. It starts with embracing body positivity. Many individuals struggle with negative body image, which can hinder their ability to enjoy solo exploration. It's essential to recognize and challenge these negative thoughts, reframing them into affirmations of self-love and appreciation for one's unique body.

Listening to one's body during exploration is crucial. Each individual has unique preferences, and understanding what feels good can take time. Tuning into bodily signals and being patient with oneself can lead to profound discoveries about pleasure and desire. Keeping a journal to reflect on experiences can also facilitate this journey, helping individuals track their thoughts and preferences over time.

As one embarks on this journey of self-exploration, an open-minded attitude is key. Embracing curiosity allows for

Ethan Wellspring

the exploration of new techniques, fantasies, and experiences. The process is not about achieving a specific goal but rather enjoying the journey itself. Solo exploration is an ever-evolving practice that can lead to greater self-discovery and, ultimately, a deeper connection with partners.

In summary, empowering solo exploration is about fostering a deeper connection with oneself, cultivating sexual self-awareness, and embracing the journey of pleasure. This chapter has outlined the significance of self-exploration, provided practical tools and techniques to enhance the experience, and emphasized the importance of building a positive relationship with one's sexual self. As we continue this exploration, the next chapter will delve into the dynamics of building a fulfilling sex life with partners, drawing on the insights gained through solo exploration.

Ethan Wellspring

Ethan Wellspring

Chapter 6: Building a Fulfilling Sex Life with Your Partner

A fulfilling sex life is a cornerstone of healthy relationships, enhancing intimacy, trust, and emotional connection. As we navigate the complexities of partnered sexuality, it's essential to understand the dynamics that contribute to a satisfying sexual relationship. This chapter delves into the vital components of building and maintaining a fulfilling sex life with your partner, emphasizing trust, vulnerability, communication, and the exploration of fantasies.

The Role of Trust and Vulnerability

Trust is the bedrock of any intimate relationship, especially when it comes to sexuality. For partners to explore their desires fully, they must feel safe and supported in their sexual experiences. Building trust involves creating an environment where both partners feel respected and valued. This requires open dialogue about feelings, preferences, and boundaries.

Ethan Wellspring

Vulnerability plays a crucial role in sexual intimacy. It allows partners to share their true selves, including their desires and insecurities. Being vulnerable fosters deeper connections and creates a space where both partners can express themselves freely without fear of judgment. When couples embrace vulnerability, they unlock new dimensions of intimacy that enhance sexual satisfaction.

Creating Emotional and Sexual Intimacy

To cultivate a fulfilling sex life, emotional intimacy is just as important as physical intimacy. Couples must prioritize emotional connections, nurturing their relationship outside the bedroom to enhance their sexual experiences. Engaging in activities that foster emotional bonding—such as sharing experiences, discussing dreams, and supporting each other through challenges—can significantly enhance sexual intimacy.

Physical touch is another critical element in building intimacy. Simple gestures like holding hands, hugging, or cuddling can create a strong emotional connection. These small acts of affection lay the groundwork for deeper

Ethan Wellspring

sexual intimacy, reinforcing feelings of love and safety between partners.

The Art of Open and Honest Sexual Communication

Communication is the linchpin of a fulfilling sex life. Open, honest conversations about sexual desires, boundaries, and preferences are essential for ensuring that both partners feel satisfied and fulfilled. Discussing fantasies, likes, and dislikes can help partners understand each other's needs, leading to more enjoyable sexual experiences.

Approaching sexual communication can be daunting, but there are effective strategies to facilitate these discussions. Setting aside dedicated time to talk about intimacy, free from distractions, can create a comfortable environment. Using "I" statements—such as "I feel" or "I would like"— can help express personal feelings without sounding accusatory, fostering a more constructive dialogue.

Navigating Differences in Libido and Desires

Ethan Wellspring

It's common for couples to experience mismatched libidos or differing sexual desires. Navigating these differences requires understanding, patience, and collaboration. Rather than viewing these disparities as obstacles, couples can approach them as opportunities for growth and connection.

Finding a compromise is key. Partners can explore various ways to meet each other's needs, whether it's scheduling intimate moments, exploring new activities together, or prioritizing quality over quantity. Understanding each partner's perspective and working together to find solutions can enhance the relationship and lead to more satisfying sexual experiences.

Exploring Fantasies Together

Exploring fantasies can be an exciting way to enhance sexual intimacy. Sharing fantasies creates an opportunity for partners to discover new aspects of each other's sexuality while deepening their connection. Engaging in this practice requires a foundation of trust and open communication.

Ethan Wellspring

When discussing fantasies, it's essential to approach the conversation with curiosity rather than judgment. Partners should feel free to express their desires without fear of rejection. This exploration can lead to exciting discoveries and new experiences, helping to keep the sexual connection alive and vibrant.

Maintaining Sexual Passion in Long-Term Relationships

As relationships evolve, it's common for sexual passion to wane over time. However, couples can take proactive steps to maintain and reignite desire. Setting aside regular date nights, prioritizing physical intimacy, and introducing novelty into the sexual routine can help keep the flame alive.

Creativity is crucial in maintaining sexual passion. Trying new activities, exploring different locations, or experimenting with new techniques can inject excitement into the relationship. Keeping the lines of communication open about desires and preferences also ensures that both partners remain engaged and invested in each other's pleasure.

Ethan Wellspring

In conclusion, building a fulfilling sex life with a partner requires effort, communication, and a commitment to understanding each other's needs. By prioritizing trust, vulnerability, emotional intimacy, and open dialogue, couples can create a rich and rewarding sexual relationship that enhances their overall connection. As we move forward, the next chapter will focus on sexual wellness and health, highlighting essential aspects of maintaining a healthy sexual life.

Ethan Wellspring

Chapter 7: Sexual Wellness and Health

Sexual wellness is an integral part of overall health and well-being. It encompasses not only the physical aspects of sexual health but also emotional, mental, and social dimensions. In this chapter, we will explore the concept of sexual wellness, the importance of sexual health for women, and the balance of mental and emotional health as they relate to intimacy and sexual experiences.

Understanding Sexual Wellness

Sexual wellness refers to a state of physical, emotional, mental, and social well-being in relation to sexuality. It goes beyond the absence of disease or dysfunction; it involves a positive and respectful approach to sexuality and sexual relationships. Understanding this holistic view of sexual wellness can empower individuals to take charge of their sexual health.

Ethan Wellspring

Several factors contribute to sexual wellness, including:

- **Knowledge and Education:** Understanding one's body, sexual health, and reproductive rights is crucial for informed decision-making and fostering a healthy sexual life.
- **Communication:** Open dialogue about sexual health, desires, and boundaries enhances intimate relationships and contributes to sexual satisfaction.
- **Consent and Respect**: A fundamental aspect of sexual wellness is ensuring that all sexual encounters are consensual and that partners respect each other's boundaries and preferences.

Promoting sexual wellness involves regular check-ups, practicing safe sex, and being aware of one's body and its needs. This awareness is vital for fostering healthy relationships and enhancing personal satisfaction.

Ethan Wellspring

Sexual Health for Women: What You Need to Know

Women's sexual health encompasses various aspects, including reproductive health, sexual function, and the management of sexually transmitted infections (STIs). It's important for women to prioritize regular check-ups with healthcare providers, which can include:

- **Routine Gynecological Exams:** Regular visits to a gynecologist for pelvic exams, Pap smears, and breast exams are essential for maintaining reproductive health.
- **Sexually Transmitted Infection (STI) Testing:** Regular STI screenings are crucial for sexually active individuals, as many STIs can be asymptomatic yet still pose serious health risks. Knowing one's status allows for prompt treatment and prevents transmission to partners.
- **Contraceptive Counseling:** Understanding birth control options and finding the right method for individual needs is vital for sexual health and family planning.

Ethan Wellspring

Additionally, hormonal changes throughout life—such as those experienced during menstruation, pregnancy, and menopause—can significantly impact sexual health. Awareness of these changes and their effects can empower women to seek appropriate medical advice and explore options that enhance sexual satisfaction.

Balancing Mental and Emotional Health

Mental and emotional health significantly impacts sexual well-being. Factors such as stress, anxiety, depression, and past trauma can influence sexual desire and function. It is essential to acknowledge these aspects and seek support when needed.

- **Stress Management:** Chronic stress can hinder sexual desire and enjoyment. Engaging in self-care practices—such as exercise, meditation, or hobbies—can alleviate stress and promote overall well-being.

Ethan Wellspring

- **Seeking Professional Help:** Therapy can be an invaluable resource for individuals struggling with mental health issues that affect their sexual lives. A therapist can provide tools and strategies for coping with anxiety, depression, or trauma, ultimately improving sexual experiences.

- **Healthy Relationships:** Building and maintaining healthy relationships with partners is key to emotional well-being. Open communication, mutual respect, and emotional support can create a safe space for intimacy to flourish.

The Intersection of Sexual and Mental Health

Research increasingly recognizes the connection between sexual health and mental health. Women who experience low sexual desire may also struggle with mental health issues, creating a cycle that can be challenging to break. Understanding this interplay is crucial for developing effective treatment plans and supportive strategies.

Ethan Wellspring

Practicing self-compassion and embracing one's sexuality can promote mental well-being. Engaging in self-reflection, exploring desires, and celebrating one's body can foster a positive mindset, leading to enhanced sexual experiences.

In summary, sexual wellness and health are vital components of a fulfilling and satisfying sexual life. By prioritizing regular health check-ups, understanding reproductive health, and addressing mental and emotional well-being, individuals can cultivate a holistic approach to their sexual health. In the next chapter, we will explore common sexual challenges women face and provide practical solutions for overcoming these obstacles.

Ethan Wellspring

Chapter 8: Navigating Sexual Challenges

Sexual challenges can arise for various reasons, impacting individuals' and couples' sexual experiences. Understanding these challenges and developing strategies to address them is essential for maintaining a fulfilling sexual life. This chapter will cover common sexual challenges women face, when to seek help, and practical solutions and exercises to overcome these obstacles.

Common Sexual Challenges Women Face

Women may encounter a range of sexual challenges, including:

- **Low Libido:** Many women experience fluctuations in sexual desire due to factors such as hormonal changes, stress, fatigue, or relationship dynamics. Low libido can lead to feelings of inadequacy and strain relationships.

Ethan Wellspring

- **Painful Sex (Dyspareunia):** Pain during intercourse can stem from various causes, including medical conditions (like endometriosis or vulvodynia), insufficient lubrication, or emotional factors like anxiety or past trauma. Understanding the root cause is crucial for finding effective solutions.

- **Difficulty Reaching Orgasm:** Many women report difficulty in achieving orgasm, which can stem from physical or psychological barriers. Factors such as stress, performance anxiety, or lack of knowledge about one's body can contribute to this challenge.

- **Body Image Issues:** Negative perceptions of one's body can hinder sexual enjoyment and intimacy. Women may feel self-conscious about their appearance, affecting their ability to engage in sexual activities fully.

Understanding these challenges is the first step towards addressing them. Recognizing that these issues are common can help alleviate feelings of isolation and shame.

Ethan Wellspring

When to Seek Help

Knowing when to seek professional help is crucial for overcoming sexual challenges. If any of the following apply, it may be time to consult a healthcare provider or a therapist:

- **Persistent Issues:** If sexual challenges persist despite efforts to address them or begin to affect your emotional well-being or relationships.

- **Physical Pain**: Experiencing pain during sex should never be ignored. Consulting a healthcare professional can help identify any underlying medical conditions.

- **Emotional Distress:** If feelings of anxiety, depression, or shame regarding sexuality become overwhelming, seeking therapy can provide valuable support and coping strategies.

Ethan Wellspring

- **Relationship Strain:** If sexual issues are causing significant stress in your relationship, couples counseling may help partners navigate their challenges together.

Professional help can offer guidance and support tailored to individual needs, making it easier to navigate sexual difficulties.

Practical Solutions and Exercises

Addressing sexual challenges often involves a combination of education, communication, and exploration. Here are practical solutions and exercises to consider:

1. Self-Exploration: Understanding your body is crucial for enhancing sexual experiences. Engage in self-exploration through masturbation, focusing on what feels pleasurable. This can help increase sexual awareness and confidence.

2. Open Communication: Discussing sexual challenges with your partner can foster understanding and intimacy. Share feelings and concerns openly, focusing on finding solutions together. Using "I" statements can help express feelings without placing blame.

3. Seek Professional Guidance: Whether it's a sex therapist, psychologist, or gynecologist, consulting a professional can provide valuable insights and tools for overcoming sexual challenges. They can also help address any underlying medical issues.

4. Experiment with Lubricants: For those experiencing pain during intercourse, using lubricants can significantly enhance comfort. Experimenting with different types of lubricants can lead to improved sexual experiences.

5. Explore New Techniques: Trying different positions, settings, or techniques can reignite sexual excitement and address issues like low libido. Introducing novelty can help partners reconnect and rediscover pleasure together.

6. Mindfulness and Relaxation: Stress and anxiety can hinder sexual enjoyment. Practicing mindfulness or relaxation techniques, such as deep breathing, yoga, or

Ethan Wellspring

meditation, can help alleviate anxiety and enhance intimacy.

7. Educate Yourself: Understanding female anatomy, sexual response, and techniques can empower women to take control of their sexual experiences. Resources like books, workshops, or online courses can provide valuable information.

8. Couples Exercises: Engaging in activities together outside the bedroom—such as dancing, cooking, or exploring new hobbies—can enhance emotional intimacy, contributing to a more fulfilling sexual relationship.

In conclusion, navigating sexual challenges is an integral part of maintaining a fulfilling sex life. By understanding common issues, knowing when to seek help, and employing practical strategies, individuals can enhance their sexual experiences and foster deeper connections with their partners. In the next chapter, we will explore the theme of sexual empowerment, focusing on how women can embrace their sexuality at different stages of life and continue their journey of self-discovery and fulfillment.

Ethan Wellspring

Chapter 9: Embracing Your Sexual Empowerment

Sexual empowerment is a journey of self-discovery, growth, and liberation. It's about understanding your body, desires, and boundaries and claiming your right to enjoy a fulfilling sexual life. In this chapter, we will redefine sexual empowerment, explore how women can embrace their sexuality at various life stages, and inspire readers to view their sexual journeys as ongoing processes of self-discovery.

Redefining Sexual Empowerment

Sexual empowerment is not just about sexual experiences; it encompasses the entire spectrum of one's relationship with sexuality. It involves:

- **Self-Confidence:** Feeling comfortable and confident in your body and desires, recognizing

Ethan Wellspring

that your sexual needs and preferences are valid and important.

- **Knowledge:** Being informed about your body, sexual health, and rights. Education can lead to better choices and experiences.

- **Communication:** Being able to express your desires and boundaries with partners openly and honestly. Communication fosters intimacy and understanding.

- **Freedom from Shame**: Letting go of societal expectations and norms that dictate what a "proper" sexual experience should be. Embracing your unique sexual identity is essential for empowerment.

- **Agency:** Taking control of your sexual experiences, making choices that align with your values, desires, and needs.

Ethan Wellspring

By redefining sexual empowerment, women can approach their sexuality with confidence and curiosity, paving the way for a more fulfilling and joyful sexual life.

Sexual Empowerment at Every Age

1. Young Adulthood: For young women, this phase often involves exploration and discovery. It's a time to learn about one's body and desires, navigate relationships, and understand the importance of consent. Engaging in open conversations about sexuality, either with trusted friends or professionals, can provide valuable insights and build a foundation for healthy sexual experiences.

2. Parenthood: Women who become mothers often face shifts in their sexual identity. Hormonal changes, body image issues, and the demands of parenting can impact sexual desire and intimacy. It's crucial for mothers to prioritize self-care, engage in open communication with partners, and embrace their evolving sexuality. Remember that a fulfilling sexual life can coexist with parenthood, and prioritizing intimacy is essential for maintaining connection.

Ethan Wellspring

3. Midlife: As women enter midlife, they may experience changes due to hormonal fluctuations, menopause, or shifts in relationship dynamics. This period often brings opportunities for self-reflection and renewal. Embracing this stage means understanding the changes in your body and finding ways to adapt and explore new avenues of pleasure. Educating yourself about sexual health and wellness during this time can empower you to make informed choices.

4. Later Life: Sexuality does not end with age; rather, it can transform and evolve. Women in their later years can still experience desire, intimacy, and pleasure. It's essential to embrace the wisdom and experience that come with age, allowing for new forms of connection and exploration. Open discussions about sexual health, relationship dynamics, and desires can enhance intimacy and fulfillment.

Ethan Wellspring

Creating a Lifelong Journey of Sexual Fulfillment

Embracing sexual empowerment is an ongoing journey. Here are some strategies to foster a lifelong connection to your sexual self:

- **Cultivate Curiosity:** Approach your sexuality with a sense of wonder and curiosity. Explore new techniques, fantasies, and experiences, whether alone or with a partner.

- **Prioritize Self-Care:** Self-care is essential for maintaining a healthy sexual life. Engage in activities that promote mental, emotional, and physical well-being.

- **Build Supportive Communities**: Seek out supportive networks, whether through friends, workshops, or online communities. Sharing experiences and insights can help normalize

Ethan Wellspring

discussions around sexuality and empower individuals to embrace their desires.

- **Stay Educated:** Continuously educate yourself about sexual health, relationships, and empowerment. Knowledge is a powerful tool for reclaiming your sexuality and ensuring a fulfilling sexual life.

- **Practice Self-Compassion:** Recognize that your sexual journey is unique, and it's okay to experience ups and downs. Practice self-compassion and forgive yourself for any perceived shortcomings.

As you navigate your journey toward sexual empowerment, remember that it's a deeply personal experience that evolves over time. Embracing your sexual self means celebrating your individuality, desires, and choices. By understanding your body and needs, you open the door to deeper connections, enhanced pleasure, and a more fulfilling sexual life.

Ethan Wellspring

In every stage of life, from youthful exploration to the wisdom of later years, embrace your sexuality with confidence and pride. Your journey is uniquely yours—one filled with the potential for discovery, joy, and empowerment. Always remember that the pursuit of sexual fulfillment is a beautiful journey worth embracing, enriching not only your life but also your relationships with others.

Conclusion

As we conclude this exploration of sexual self-awareness and empowerment, it's essential to recognize that embracing your sexuality is a lifelong journey filled with discovery, growth, and fulfillment. Throughout this book, we have unpacked the various dimensions of sexual self-awareness, body positivity, communication, and intimacy, guiding you toward a more empowered relationship with your sexual self.

Ethan Wellspring

The Path Forward:

The key lessons from this journey include the importance of understanding your body, nurturing self-confidence, and fostering open communication with partners. Overcoming societal taboos, addressing sexual challenges, and exploring intimacy at various life stages are vital components of this journey. Remember that your sexual identity is not static; it evolves with you, shaped by your experiences, desires, and the ongoing pursuit of knowledge.

Embrace the freedom to explore, express, and enjoy your sexuality fully. Be proactive in seeking support, educating yourself, and celebrating your desires. The journey of sexual empowerment is yours to define, and by embracing it, you can cultivate a fulfilling, joyful, and vibrant sexual life.

As you move forward, carry with you the understanding that sexual empowerment is not just a destination; it's a continuous journey of self-discovery, growth, and love. Embrace your sexual self, honor your desires, and take

Ethan Wellspring

pride in the beautiful, complex, and ever-evolving nature
of your sexuality.

Ethan Wellspring